# Henna

## The Environmentally Friendly Way to Colour Your Hair

## A Step-by-Step Guide to Apply Henna

By Daisy Green

# Other books by Daisy Green

The Sleep fairy

Leo and the Sleep Fairy

Noah and The Sleep Fairy

George and The Sleep Fairy

*For a healthy environment*

First published by CreateSpace for and on
behalf of theyellowmoon.com, a wholly owned
subsidiary of Daisy Green.

This edition published in 2016
by CreateSpace, USA
Associated companies throughout the world.

ISBN-10: 1530098580

# Henna

The Environmentally Friendly
Way to Colour Your Hair

A Step-by-Step Guide
to Apply Henna

By Daisy Green

# Contents

# Introduction

Henna is a natural product, taken from a plant called Lawsonia Inermis.

Henna grows in dry regions, mostly in Middle-Eastern and southern Asian countries such as India, where climate is arid and temperature is generally above 20 degrees.

There is evidence in history that women have been using Henna since about 3000 years before Christ and possibly even earlier. Over the centuries, and in some places, Henna is still being used for medicinal purposes, for painting fingernails, the soles of the feet, face, hands as well as hair.

You can get many types of Henna in the shops. Many types have added colour, chemicals or other ingredients. But from my experience, I found that most of those were not as good as the natural organic Henna that I found. This recipe I developed over two years of experimenting and making notes. I decided to share it with you because there was not enough information available on preparing and applying Henna.

I kept the details and instructions in this book as simple as possible, because I am sure that you just want to have beautiful hair, without any mess.

# About the Author

I grew up in Africa, where everything I put on my hair and skin was natural and organic.

After spending years in the west, and becoming accustomed to advertising, I felt compelled to bleach my hair, dye it, straighten it and so on. I tried everything to look the part, to look like the girls on TV, in magazines and on the street.

Eventually, I discovered that all that we put on our hair makes it dry, damaged, thin and frizzy. It needs more treatments and more chemicals. The cycle goes on.

I stopped putting any chemicals on my hair. But when I reached my late 30's, grey hair began to show and quickly became very obvious. My hair became more dry, wiry, frizzy and dull looking.

People kept saying: 'oh you should dye your hair'. 'You mustn't go out like this'. 'Don't let the grey show' etc. So I returned to my roots and to nature. This is one of many books to come, to treat our body with care: to change hair colour without hurting it.

For two years I tried and tested different ingredients. I kept a diary until a recipe emerged that worked well. I decided to share it with you.

# A Note Before You Start

Please remember these are guidelines, and the first time for everything is a little tricky, so have faith; your second time will be even better.

Also, please note that you are responsible for checking if an ingredient may cause you allergy or undesirable reaction. I have tried and tested the ingredients in this recipe. Now you must do that for yourself too.

Your hair type may be different to mine. My hair is dark with some grey and some highlights. It is fine and dry. If your hair is oily or blonde, for example, use this recipe as a guideline; test the ingredients and adjust the recipe to your specific hair needs.

Also, I recommend that you read through the whole book before you start applying the Henna. So here we go!

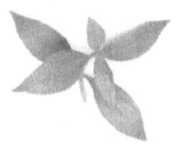

# Where to Get the Best Henna

There are many shops and websites where you can get Henna. The best Henna, from my experience is one that has not been mixed for you, it should be organically certified, fine and pure. The packet's ingredients should say 100% pure Henna.

I have tried Henna others from different outlets. But found some types were mixed, dry and even sandy. One packet I bought in a shop made my hair feel like wooden strands.

I live in the UK so I buy my Henna from Neal's Yard Remedies:

http://www.nealsyardremedies.com

They have stores all over Britain or you can order from them online. It's organic, pure, fine and lovely. Neal's' Yard Henna has been the best one for my hair type.

# Why Avoid Chemical Dyes

There are hundreds of types of hair dye out there, some even claim to be natural, organic or full of fruits of heaven.

All you need to do is look at the ingredients. You will see that it includes one or two extracts or a hint of a natural product and the rest are chemicals. Harmful chemicals.

Everything you put on your scalp, which is skin with thousands of hair follicles, gets ingested into your body, letting your organs struggle to deal with the toxins, some of which may linger in your body for years, causing damage that you don't want!

These are toxins. You only need to Google one to find an array of websites and information about the negative effects these chemicals have on your body.

These chemicals are harmful to our planet.

Whatever your reasons to colour your hair, why not do it without hurting your body or our planet?

# Why Use Henna

Henna is 100% natural. You can get it organic. It grows as a plant. It has been tested for centuries.

It has been used as medicine and as body art. In the ancient times, it was used to dye the hair and fur of loved animals and pets too!

All the ingredients that you can add to the recipe in this book, are natural and from your own kitchen.

Henna is an environmentally safe method of colouring hair, including all the additional ingredients that are suggested here.

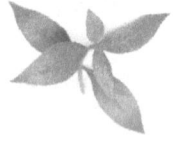

# Dark Hair

The natural colour of my hair is dark chestnut. The recipe I have developed gives me tones of deep copper red. The highlights that I have appear warm, copper. But the tone remains for up to 6 weeks or until I add more Henna to my hair.

Please note, I have chosen to make my Henna mixture to have red tones in it because I like red. But you can adjust the mixture if you prefer it to be just brown.

Henna has no bleaching properties; therefore, it will not reduce or lighten the colour of your hair, although, dark hair will have a luxurious brown or red glow in bright light or sunshine.

If you have naturally fair, blonde, red or light brown hair, I recommend that you follow the instructions but use a little personal judgement on how much red you want your hair to be. The Henna will be brighter on lighter hair.

By following my recipe as a guideline, this will be your experiment.

# Grey Hair

I have a lot of grey hair. This is what motivated me to find the most natural way to cover grey.

The recipe you're holding in your hands covers grey. It is not a 100% cover. I would say about 90%. So my dark hair shines with deep copper, and in some areas, I have streaks that are almost red. All hair tones become a warm copper/brown.

It blends in with the rest of the hair, showing natural tones of lighter and darker streaks all over. People have not been able to tell that I had grey hair before applying Henna.

That's different to chemical hair dye, which covers everything like doll's hair, despite the streaking technology and more chemicals.

If you have mainly grey hair, I recommend avoiding using beetroot all together, unless you want to have red hair. You will still get a warm brown result. It's worth experimenting with leaving the Henna on for longer.

Remember that grey hair is natural. So if you add Henna, your hair will have natural streaks of different tones of browns, coppers and reds. That's natural too.

# Highlighted or Bleached Hair

I have used Henna on my naturally dark hair, which had highlights in it.

My hairdresser confirmed that the highlighted sections in my hair would be fine with natural Henna.

If your hair is bleached, you will definitely get a bright red or orange colour. I have not experienced this and cannot advise you on it.

If you have bleached hair and would like to try Henna, I recommend that you speak to your hairdresser and do a test strand first.

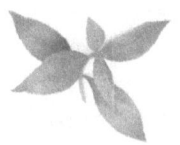

# Hair Types

I have dry, fine hair.
Please note this recipe is for dry hair.

If you have oily or normal hair, as advised earlier, please be the judge on how much olive oil to add. As you make your notes, you will prefect the recipe to suit your hair type. Use this is a guide.

Also, it will work better if you wash your hair beforehand with a mild shampoo (but no conditioner.)

The oil amount I recommend in the recipe is minimal to blend the ingredients and keep your hair soft and moisturised.

When you shampoo, any oil will wash out. If your hair is oily, it may need a second shampoo, but I don't recommend too much washing when the Henna is still fresh in the hair. No harm will come from waiting till the next day to shampoo. The Henna will get a chance to settle in its colour.

Do a strand test to see which oil suits you best. I recommend using an oil in any case, to avoid the rest of ingredients drying your hair.

# The Best Oil You Can Use

Light or Extra Virgin Olive Oil:

I found that each oil make is also different.

After trying out a few types of olive oil, I found that Filippo Berio Extra Virgin Olive oil is the most suited to my dry, fine hair.

It is natural plant oil. As you know, Olive oil is used in food recipes all around the world, so you can be sure it is safe.

You may like to tray a strand test of light olive oil if your hair is oily. Whichever one you choose will not harm your hair or scalp.

If you have allergies, please do your own tests to check before using them.

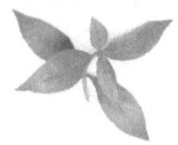

# Items You Need to Before You Start

- A packet of baby wipes and tissues for emergency drips.
- Vaseline to apply around hairline.
- A button front old top to wear during and after application, preferably dark coloured.
- An old towel to pin over shoulders while applying henna. Or a hair colouring cape.
- A large mirror.
- Prepare a clear space of at least 1-meter square for this.
- You need a bin bag open to drop things in/excess henna, tissues etc.
- Disposable shower cap ready to apply. You can order them on Amazon.
- Latex gloves (must not be loose). You can order a packet of these on Amazon.
- An old towel to towel-dry hair after rinsing henna.
- A large glass bowl, similar to one you use for making cake mixture.
- Avoid distractions: children, pets, doorbell, visitors, outings etc.
- Avoid activities that require wearing glasses!

# The Ingredients You Need for The Recipe

- Organic henna for hair. 100g for this recipe. (For medium and long hair). Less for short hair.
- For intense red results: you need organic beetroot juice or organic beetroot that you can liquidise in the blender with other ingredients.
- Organic apple cider vinegar
- Lemon juice squeezed from half a fresh lemon.
- Warm water
- For moisturising effects add extra virgin olive oil.

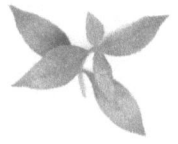

# Where is Best to Apply Henna

- Over the bathroom sink.
- In the garden if weather allows. Henna and all the ingredients are natural and the ground will soak them in.
- If you apply indoors, choose a floor that is not carpeted. If not, cover with black bin bags or plastic upside down table cloth to protect the carpet from staining.
- In front of a wall mirror if possible, with a table to put the glass bowl and other items.

# Time: From Preparation to Finish

If you apply during daytime:

- Make the mixture in an evening, so you can leave it to settle.
- Clear a day for applying henna and staying at home.
- Apply in the morning.
- Activities that require glasses will be impossible as you don't want to get your frame covered in henna.
- Wash out in the evening. Towel dry. Shampoo the following day and style.

If you apply overnight:

- Prepare rest of mixture in the morning.
- Apply in the evening.
- Use pillow protector.
- Wash out in the morning.

# Here is How I Do It

Evening of Day One:

Wash hair with normal shampoo.
Do not condition. Do not add any products.
Dry naturally.
Make the mixture in the glass bowl.
Cover it with cling film. Leave overnight.

Morning of Day Two:

Prepare the space to apply the henna mixture.
Apply mixture as per instructions.
Leave it for at least 5 hours or more.

Evening of Day Two:

Remove the mixture.
Rinse with just-warm water.
Do not shampoo or condition.
Towel-dry your hair.
Use pillow protector to avoid staining.

Morning of Day Three:

Shampoo and condition hair as normal, in warm – not hot – water.

Style as normal.

# Making The Recipe

Put the ingredients together. If you're using actual beetroots, then liquidise them first with lemon and vinegar.

Add the rest of the ingredients.

Mix well with a spoon.

Don't worry about thickness at this stage, just good mixing. The lemon will help the dye to be released from the Henna powder. Beetroot will add redness. Vinegar will add shine.

Cover with cling film. Leave in a dark place in room temperature overnight.

When you are ready to apply the Henna mixture:

Add 3 - 4 tablespoons of olive oil
Add warm water gradually to the consistency of thick yoghurt or humous. Any thinner than yogurt and you will have runny, messy Henna everywhere. Warm water is better for hair.

# How To Apply

- Make sure hair has no products on it.
- Wet and towel dry hair beforehand. No dripping. Comb it so no knots.
- Wear your gloves.
- Start where there is the most grey. Take a small amount, the size of a £2 coin, rub it on both palms.
- Take a small section of hair and apply.
- Apply from front to back. Scalp to tip.
- If your hair is long, lay every strand you cover over the top of your head, so at the end, there will be no hair over your neck.
- Keep doing this until you feel you have covered all the hair and scalp.
- If the mixture is like yoghurt or thicker, it will hold without a hairclip.
- Add any extra mixture to your head or any missed gaps, press gently to make sure every hair is covered.
- Cover your hair with cling film.
- Use baby wipes to wipe off any excess Henna that has run down the face or neck. Dispose in the bin bag, not toilet!
- As a quick action, use baby wipes to wipe any henna stains from floor/sink/wall area.
- Put all any clothing/ material in washing machine straight away to save them from staining.

# Washing Out The Henna

- Make sure you have the old towel to hand.
- Hold your head over the open bin bag in case of falling Henna. Gently remove the shower cap.
- Feel with your fingers, if any pieces are loose; let them fall into the bag.
- Step under warm (not hot), running shower water.
- As gently as you can, with fingers, nudge the hair, letting Henna run in the water.
- Do this as slowly and gently as possible.
- Rinse until water runs completely clear.
- With your fingers gently feel all over your scalp to make sure any excess Henna has been washed off.
- If you can resist, do not shampoo.
- Towel dry.
- Gently comb/ brush your hair.
- Use a pillow protector and old pillowcase to protect from any staining.
- Leave overnight.
- In the morning shampoo and condition as normal with warm water.
- Enjoy.

# Henna Aftercare

- Always wash hennaed hair with warm water. Never hot water as it washes out the henna too soon.

- When you wash your hennaed hair, use gentle shampoo and conditioner.

- Wash as little as you can. I wash my hair every other day.

- Once hair has henna in it, you mustn't use chemical hair dye for a good few months. Please check with your hairdresser if want to do that.

- Henna can be topped up as often as you like. I use it on average every 6 weeks, just enough to cover the new grey. But you can use it more often to keep your hair looking vibrant and shiny. It's natural after all.

- As you will note from my diary, try not leave 6 weeks between Henna applications. This will keep it topped up, so you're always adding moisture, colour and tone to the henna that's' still on your hair. Also, you get to avoid having new grey hair showing.

# Keep a Diary

To start with, I recommend keeping a diary of notes to remind yourself of what you did last time you applied henna, and if there was anything you'd like to do differently. This is how I managed to improve my recipe until I got it to how I liked it best. You can do this to get the mixture to suit your hair type, get best colour consistency that you like, and, most importantly, to find the schedule that works best for your life style.

In the next few pages, you can see part of my Henna diary as an example.

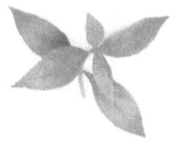

# An Extract From my Henna Diary

*1<sup>st</sup> application:*

**Kept henna on hair from 10.30am - 8.30pm**

*Result copper on grey hair. Red tones all over. Very soft. I didn't condition just shampoo and towel dry.*

*2 weeks later:*
*Grey hair still warm copper*
*Hot water washed the henna out too soon. Lost its shine, but brown tone still there.*
*New grey showing after 6 weeks.*

**6 weeks later: 12.30 to 5pm**

*Followed all above instructions, though used a glass measurement instead of spoon, mixture was a little thinner than yoghurt, so more difficult to keep on hair.*

*Rinsed with lukewarm water.*
*Shampoo but no conditioner.*

*Next time:*
*Add 3 tablespoons of olive oil.*

### *6 weeks later: 12pm to 5pm*

*It lasted much better this time, my hair is still reddish copper over grey and rest was reddish brown and shiny.*

*Added 3 table spoons of olive oil*
*Added a little warm water until it was as thick as yogurt.*

*Mixture was perfect, all stayed on hair, covered all scalp with it, pressed in tight, and covered with cap. It was warm because of the warm water, now it's warm under cap - very nice.*

*Results: the grey turned an extra hint of red.*
*My hair feels very moisturised. Rinsed with lukewarm water only. No shampoo.*

*Try shampoo next day.*

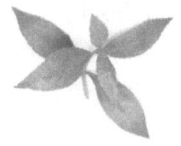

### 8 weeks later: 9.30 – 2.30pm

*The hennaed part of the hair has grown out, as left it too long, so new grey showing.*

*But the red is still strong on the hennaed grey hair from last time; even the dark (non grey) hair still shines a reddish/brown. Good progress.*

*I shampooed hair as normal night before. No conditioner.*

*Made mixture as above, with no olive oil until tomorrow. Left by radiator to keep warm over night. Washed out, no shampoo or conditioner till next day.*

### 11 weeks later: 11.45 – 5.30pm

*My hair has grown about 1inch with new grey. The rest of hair still has red in it!*

*Have highlights in hair. In the morning I added 4 spoons of olive oil and a bit of hot water to mixture. Applied as above.*
*All the grey turned brown/red. The rest is a nice rich tone.*

### 7 weeks later: 5pm - 11pm

*Mixed as original recipe*
*Added 1 full lemon*
*11 spoons of vinegar*
*11 spoons of beetroot juice*
*Left by radiator overnight*
*Shampooed and towel dried hair, no conditioner.*

*Next day:*

*I added 4 spoons of olive oil*
*Added warm water until the mixture was a bit thicker than yogurt. The olive oil made it bind together so well. There were no drips, no crumbling. No mess.*

*I managed to section my hair, and lift up a little bit with three fingers and apply slowly. I applied all of it. It looked and acted like clay. The hair stayed where I layered it over my head. It itched quite a bit to start with, but all ingredients are natural so didn't worry and it settled after a short time.*
*Rinsed in warm water only.*

*Next morning: shampooed and conditioned.*

*Hair is shiny, soft and red. The grey is copper/brown! But the general outlook is nice, with natural looking, vibrant tones.*

### *6 weeks later: 10 – 5pm*

*I decided to try something different.*

*Left hair unwashed and dry*

*I used only half a lemon in a separate bowl.*
*Added vinegar generously, leaving enough thickness to add warm water later.*

*I liquidised two organic beetroot bulbs together. Then added 4 spoons of olive oil and Henna.*

*At the end, I added warm water to get the thickness to thick yogurt/ humous consistency.*

*Left it to settle for an hour then applied as per instructions in previous pages. It worked a treat. My hair is luscious, shiny brown. All grey is covered.*

*There was no itching – so half a lemon is enough!*

So you see, these are guidelines. Now that you have everything at your fingertips, you can find your perfect henna recipe by using your diary.

# Your Diary

I recommend that you keep a Henna diary, this way you can make changes to the recipe until you get it to the perfection that suits your hair type and schedule.

Use mine as a guide.

Hair colour since last Henna:

Date of applying Henna

Time left henna on hair:

Next time add more:

Next time add less:

......

Results 6 weeks later:

New changes:

# Thank You for Purchasing This Book

I hope this information has been helpful to you and encourages you and many more women and men to use henna rather than industrial, factory made chemical dyes.

Please look out for our next book. There will be a number of these to follow. They are all about taking care of our body and hair without chemicals, without hurting the environment.

If you have used the recipe and developed your own version of it, I would be so grateful if you leave feedback on Amazon to encourage other men and women who'd like to use Henna.

Your comments and views are valuable to us, so please feel free to get in touch.

Daisy Green is part of theyellowmoon.com blog. You can reach her there, or by email on:
info@theyellowmoon.com

Please leave your feedback, your views, or share your experience on Amazon.

Good luck and let me know what happens!

Daisy Green

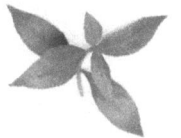

www.ingramcontent.com/pod-product-compliance
Lightning Source LLC
Chambersburg PA
CBHW030550290526
45786CB00004B/1945